Practice Technique

FRCS ORTHOPAEDICS

Clinical Examination

Subeditors

Ike Nwachukwu

Ravi Dimri

M Faisal

F R Hashmi

MBBS, BSc, FRCS Ed, FRCS T&O

Fellow Of The European Board Of Orthopaedics & Traumatology

First published in Great Britain as a softback original in 2014

Copyright © F R Hashmi

The moral right of this author has been asserted.

Typeset in Mercury

Editing, design and publishing by UK Book Publishing

UK Book Publishing is a trading name of Consilience Media

www.ukbookpublishing.com

ISBN: 978-1-910223-13-0

Dedication

For Raheel, Zeshan, Rashida and my parents

Acknowledgements

In turning this book from an idea into a reality, I am grateful to M Faisal, Peter Binfield and Ike Nwachukwu.

I would like to thank Caroline Samouelle, Jacqui Farrington and Marie Ritson for their continued support and help in providing me time and space to work on improving training and education.

I also appreciate the help of Alison Williams and Ruth Hinds from CETA Health along with Mary Calcutt and Jordan Lott from SWFT who helped me with organising and compiling the images used in this book. Also thanks to Michelle Powell who modelled for the pictures.

My secretary Verity Cox and Hayley Ellis who worked tirelessly to put my words into writing, need special thanks.

I must not forget to mention my senior peers Peter Millner, David Macdonald and Abhay Rao from Leeds and David Wise and Ravi Dimri from Huddersfield for the help and guidance in shaping up my career and teaching skills.

Last but not the least my wife Rashida and boys Zeshan and Raheel.

Contributors

Mr Ike Nwachukwu FRCS Eng, FRCS (Tr and Orth)

Chairman and Head of Training Department of Orthopaedics
Consultant Orthopaedic Surgeon & Senior Upper Limb Specialist
Shoulder and Hip Sports Surgery, UK

Mr P M Binfield FRCS (Orth)

Consultant Orthopaedic Surgeon, UK
Warwick Hospital
South Warwickshire NHS Foundation Trust

Mr K Shah FRCS, MBMS, M.Ch (Tr and Orth)

Consultant Orthopaedic Surgeon, UK
Warwick Hospital
South Warwickshire NHS Foundation Trust

Mr J Waite FRCS (Orth)

Consultant Orthopaedic Surgeon, UK
Warwick Hospital
South Warwickshire NHS Foundation Trust

Mr M Faisal FRCS Ed (Tr and Orth), MRcs, Msc, M.S (Ortho)

Consultant Orthopaedic Surgeon, UK
Warwick Hospital
South Warwickshire NHS Foundation Trust

Mr R Sloan FRCS (Tr and Orth)

Consultant Orthopaedic Surgeon
Shoulder and Upper Limb Specialist, UK
Warwick Hospital
South Warwickshire NHS Foundation Trust

Mr Amjad Shad FRCS Ed, FRCS (SN)

Consultant Neurosurgeon, UK
University Hospital Coventry and Warwickshire NHS Trust

Prof. Dr. med. Dr. H. C. Edgar Mayr

Head of Department
Professor of Surgery, Orthopaedics and Traumatology
Klinikum Augsburg, Germany

Prof. Habib Rahman MBBS, FRCS (Ortho), FCPS (orthopaedics)

Heart of England NHS Foundation Trust
Birmingham, UK

Dr Jameel Ahmad Khan MBBS, RMP

Clinical Director
Tariq Hospital
Fazilpur, Pakistan

Talat Bashir Khan BSc, MBBS, FRCS

Professor Orthopaedic Surgery
Avicenna Medical College
Lahore, Pakistan

Ravinder K Dimri FRCS (Tr and Orth)

Consultant Orthopaedic Surgeon
Huddersfield Royal Infirmary
Calderdale & Huddersfield NHS Foundation Trust

Foreword

The examination of a patient is based on three pillars:

Taking the history of a patient, the clinical examination and the examination with technical support.

We all are trained especially to read, for example, X-rays, CT-scans or MRI-scans, which are the technical examinations. A real education in clinical examination is lacking in many cases; an education in how to evaluate the history of a patient is not trained at all in most cases.

This new book by Mr Hashmi therefore gives an excellent overview about how to evaluate the history of a patient and it is a perfect overview of the most important clinical testings for the most common orthopaedic disorders one gets to see on a daily basis. When you have read this book and you have trained to perform the clinical examinations, readers will have knowledge about the suffering of their patients before technical examinations are done. Therefore this book is an excellent, perfectly structured aid, especially for young doctors who want to develop a routine in the clinical examination of patients.

Prof. Dr. med. Dr. H. C. Edgar Mayr

Head of Department

Professor of Surgery, Orthopaedics and Traumatalogy

Klinikum Augsburg

Germany

Preface

Orthopaedic trainees should find this book useful early in their clinical careers and heading for professional exams.

The book was developed to accompany FRCS (Orthopaedics) revision courses which are held at this institution.

We have used the feedback of our teaching to refine the book's content and common sense approach.

Clinical exams are stressful and clear guidance in a simple format can aid performance under these conditions.

A book is no substitute to seeing patients and 'hands on' teaching but can give us valuable support.

Peter Binfield

Consultant Orthopaedic Surgeon

Warwick Hospital, Warwickshire

Contents

History
Taking

History

Taking history from the patient is an art and candidates have limited time, in FRCS examination – a maximum of five minutes is allotted for history taking in intermediate cases.

With a few modifications the main points are similar during the history taking of different joints problems. I have tried to summarise these points with four headings: pain; other symptoms; effects on daily activities; and past history. These four headings can easily be changed to the relevant case examination.

Pain:

- where
- when
- how long
- radiation
- type
- nocturnal
- aggravating and relieving factors
- start up pain

Other Symptoms:

- stiffness
- deformity
- give-way
- locking
- spine (numbness, weakness, bowel or bladder problems and weight loss)

Effect on daily activities:

Hip	Knee
walking supports	locking
walking distance	swelling
using stairs	giving way
cutting toenails	deformity
using transport	

Past history:

- previous treatment
- injury
- surgery in the past
- similar episodes

An example

Knee examination History

1. ODP: Origin, Duration and Progress

How did the pain start, how long has it been going on and how it has progressed to present position?

2. ADL (Activities of daily living):

How does it affect your activities of daily living like walking, climbing stairs, night pain and your hobbies?

3. What treatment have you had so far, eg: physiotherapy, pain killers and injections?

How effective has the treatment been?

4. What is your quality of life because of the knee pain – has it deteriorated?

5. Have you got any mechanical symptoms like:

- knee locking, giving way or clicking?
- hip – start up pain, walking?
- spine – pain on moving, bowel and bladder problem, weight loss?

What activities make it give way or lock and how do you unlock it?

Personal and Social History:

- Do you live in a house or bungalow?
- Smoking?
- Alcohol?

Past Medical History:

Do you suffer from any serious heart or chest problem or any medical condition like hypertension, diabetes?

Did you have any surgery in the past? If it was orthopaedic treatment then ask how effective previous THR (total hip replacement) or TKR has been.

Do you suffer from any back trouble? If yes, ask for neurological symptoms.

Present Medical Treatment:

Anti hypertensive, diabetic medicine, warfarin and allergy to any drugs or artificial materials

Now specific points for each region's history taking:

Hip

- For how long have you had the symptoms?
- Walking distance: Yards / minutes
- Sleep disturbance
- Painkillers
- Effect on daily activities of living eg:
- stairs, washing, dressing, getting in and out of a chair/Car, etc
- What treatment have you had to date?

Past medical history:

- Cardiovascular
- Diabetes
- Smoking
- Surgical procedures
- DVT/CVA

Allergies:

- Drugs
- Food
- Metal eg Nickel

Knee

1. **ODP: Origin, Duration and Progress**

How did the pain start, how long has it been going on and how has it progressed to present position?

2. **ADL: How does it affect your activities of daily living like walking, climbing stairs, night pain and your hobbies?**

3. **What treatment did you have so far, eg physiotherapy, pain killers and injections?**

How effective has the treatment been?

4. **What is your quality of life because of the knee pain? Has it deteriorated?**

5. **Have you got any mechanical symptoms like knee locking, giving way or clicking?**

What activities make it give way or lock and how do you unlock it?

Personal and Social History:

- Do you live in a house or bungalow?
- Smoking
- Alcohol

Past Medical History:

- Do you suffer from any serious heart or chest problem or any medical condition like hypertension, diabetes?

- Did you have any surgery in the past? If it was orthopaedic treatment then ask how effective previous Arthroscopy, THR OR TKR has been.

- Do you suffer from any back trouble? If yes, ask for neurological symptoms.

Present Medical Treatment:

Anti hypertensive, diabetic medicine, warfarin and allergy to any drugs or artificial materials

Shoulder

Hand dominance

ODP:

Pain

Other symptoms:

- Stiffness
- Instability (popping out of shoulder)

ADL:

- Hair combing
- Putting / taking off shirt
- Doing and undoing the bra
- Sporting activity

Past history:

- Similar episode in the past
- Previous treatment, eg physiotherapy, injections, surgery

Spine

ODP (Onset, Duration, Progress of symptoms)

Pain

- Where (leg vs back)
- When
- Radiation
- Type
- Nocturnal
- Aggravating/ relieving factors

Other Symptoms

- Stiffness
- Deformity
- Numbness
- Weakness
- Bladder and bowel
- Weight loss
- Scoliosis (when, how, progression, pain, neurobiological symptoms, growth, menarche, family history, previous treatment)

Functional history

ADL (Activities of Daily Living)

- Walking
- Limp
- Support
- Distance

- Stairs
- Transport

Past history

- Injury
- Treatment
- Surgery
- Similar episodes

Notes

Clinical Examination

Intermediate
Cases

Intermediate Cases

In the FRCS Examination there are two intermediate cases. Allow 15 minutes for each: during each case 5 minutes for history taking, 5 minutes for examination and 5 minutes for discussion about the case management.

When candidates stay within the allotted time frame it becomes easier and less stressful.

During clinical examination follow the routine of:

Look

Feel

Move

Special tests

Hip examination

Introduce yourself to the patient; ask permission for the examination.

Look around for walking aid, inserts or built-up shoes or prosthesis.

Gait

Try to recognise the Type (ie Trendelenburg, Antalgic, Shuffling, Waddling) – otherwise describe the walk with normal gait (heel to toe gait).

Trendelenburg test

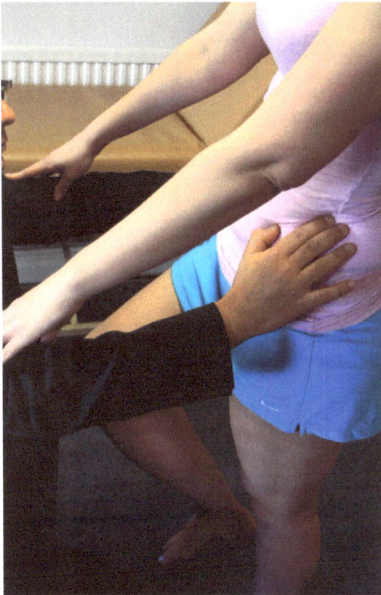

Kneel, facing the patient. Place your hands on the patient's anterior superior iliac spines with the patient resting their hands on your shoulders. Ask the patient to stand on their bad leg with the good leg flexed at the knee– this will cause a drooping of the pelvis on the opposite side from the horizontal plane (sound side sags) due to inefficiency of the abductor mechanism and you will feel increased pressure on your hand on the affected side.

A positive test can be due to inefficiency of the abductor muscles, pain, CDH, gross coxa vara, post polio and post THR exposure.

Lying down

- Look and confirm the inspection finding.
- Square the pelvis.

Leg length measurement

Apparent leg length
From xephisternum to medial maleolus

True leg length (with the pelvis squared)
From anterior superior iliac spine to medial maleolus

Depending upon presence of shortening check Bryant's Triangle to rule out proximal shortening

Bryant's Triangle

A line is drawn vertically downward from the ASIS. Another line from the ASIS to the tip of the greater trochanter and lastly a horizontal line from the tip of the greater trochanter to the first line. Diminution of the horizontal line in comparison to the opposite side denotes proximal migration of the trochanter eg in transcervical or subcapital fracture neck of femur or slipped capital femoral epiphysis.

Diminution or increase in the second line indicates the anterior or posterior displacement of the trochanter accordingly (anterior or posterior dislocation of the hip respectively).

Thomas test

With the patient lying flat on a couch, flex the affected hip as far as it will go (comment on the range). Place your hand under the small of the patient's back. Ask the patient to flex the non-affected side till the lumbar lordosis is obliterated. Now ask the patient to extend the affected hip and the fixed flexion deformity will become apparent, and can be noted.

Normal range of flexion is 120 degrees.

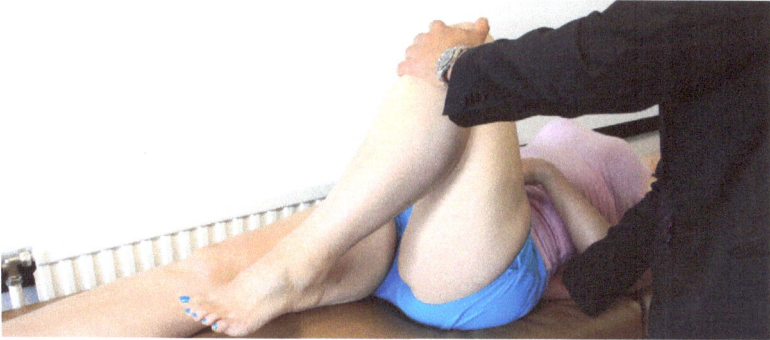

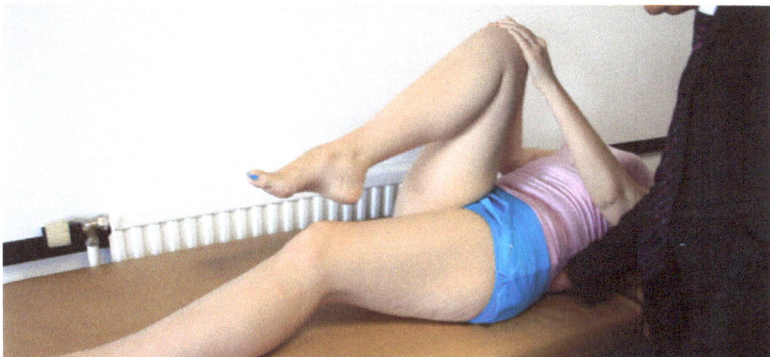

Feel

Greater trochanter, anterior superior iliac spine, anterior tenderness

Move

Abduction - (Normal range 0-45)

Adduction - (Normal range 0-45)

Rotation

Internal rotation - (Normal range 0-40)

External rotation - (Normal range 0-20)

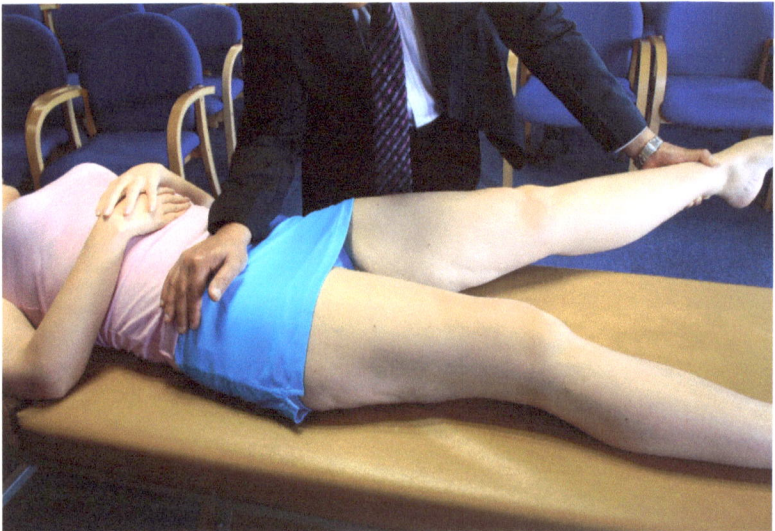

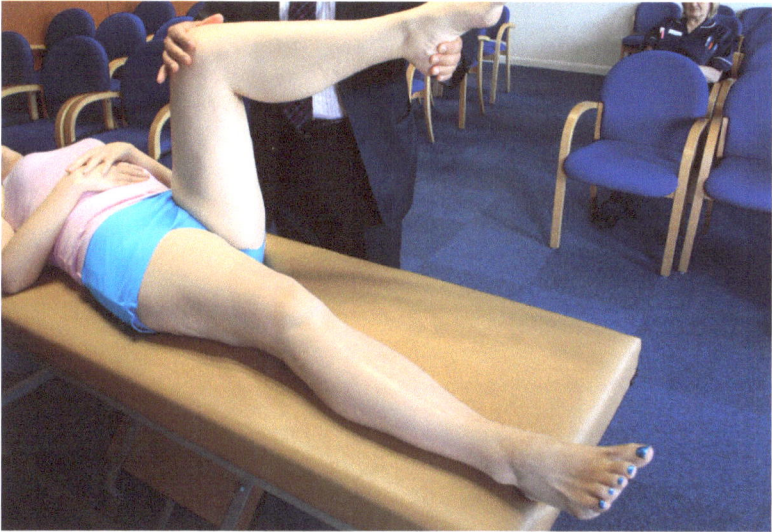

On Side

Extension

Neurovascular status

Finally mention that you will examine Back and Knee.

Knee examination

Introduce yourself to patient. Proper exposure is important so ask permission for examination.

Look around for brace, walking aid and check for wear pattern in the shoes.

Gait

Look for normal heel to toe gait. Look for varus thrust. Is it antalgic?

Look

Front
- Swelling, surgical scars, alignment and rotation
- Overall alignment when standing
- Look for increased varus or valgus
- Patella position – squinting
- Q angle

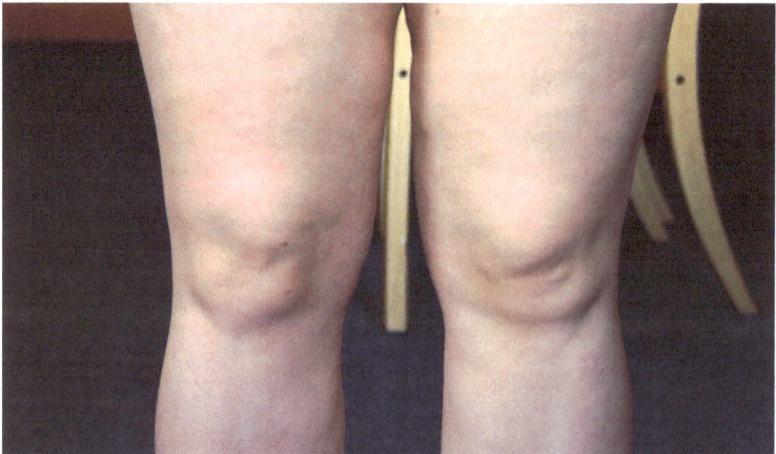

Side

- Assess patella position
- Hyperextension or fixed flexion
- Look for planovalgus feet influencing position of knee

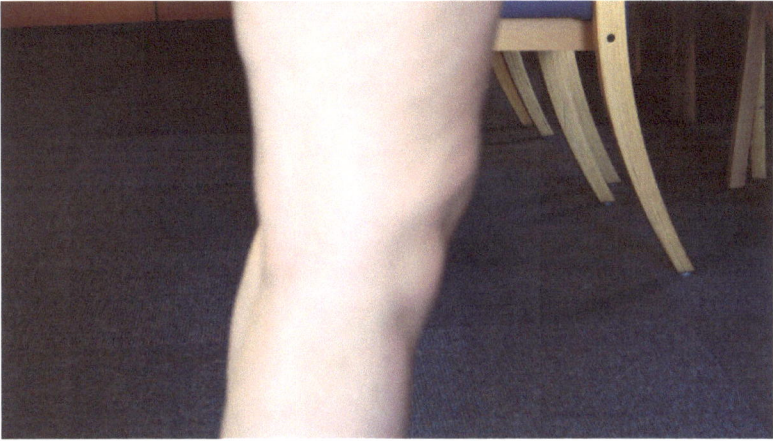

Back

- Fullness in popliteal fossa
- Calf wasting
- Heel alignment

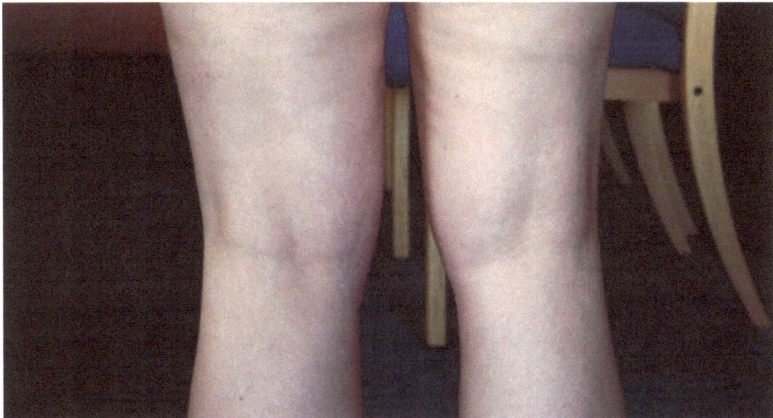

Feel

Lying down

- Look for alignment and rotational deformity
- Quantify effusion (Sweep test, balloting)
- Assess patella mobility by quadrants
- Feel for patella tilt. Is there patella irritability?
- Palpate for tender areas, especially joint lines, patella tendon, patella, ligament insertions

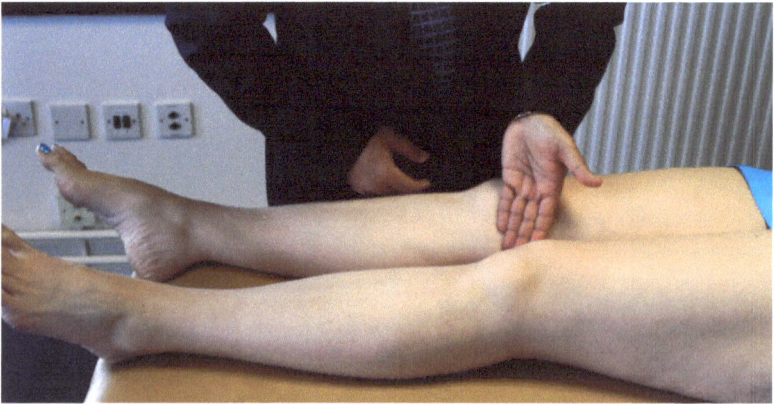

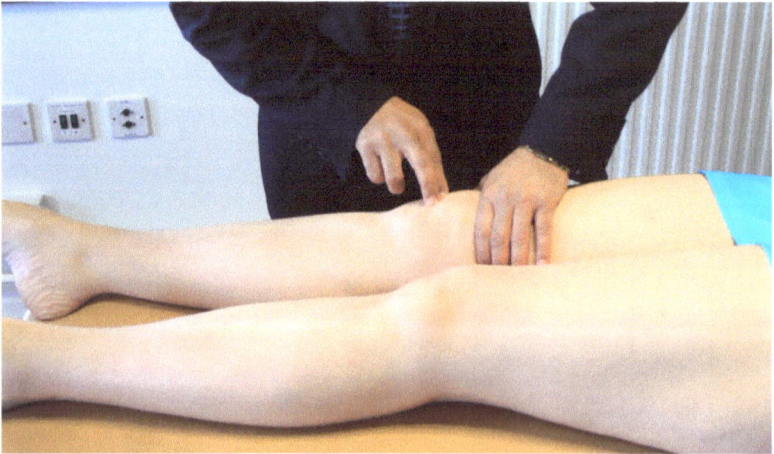

Move

- Range of movement. Check hyperextension.
- Compare with the other side.
- Check for fixed flexion deformity.
- Difference in passive and active range of movement. Is it painful?
- Feel for patella crepitus during active extension.
- Assess varus and valgus movement by stressing collateral ligaments.

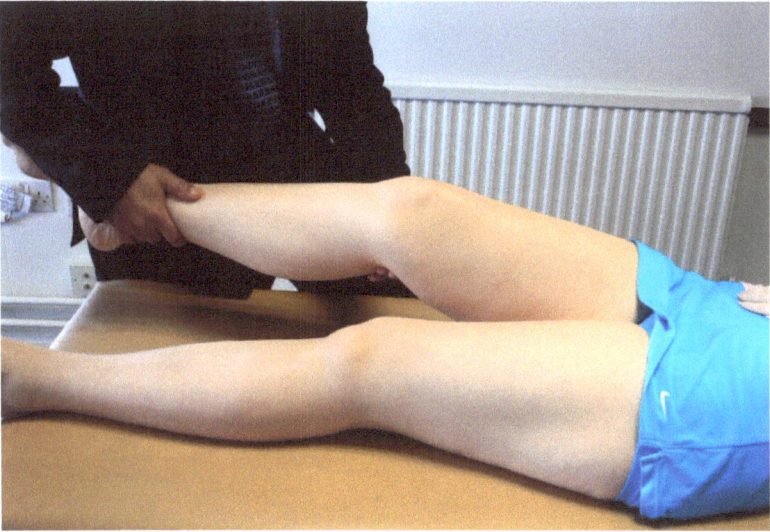

Is there laxity? Is there a solid end-point? Is it painful?

Special test

Meniscus – McMurray's test

ACL – AP glide, Lachman's, Pivot shift

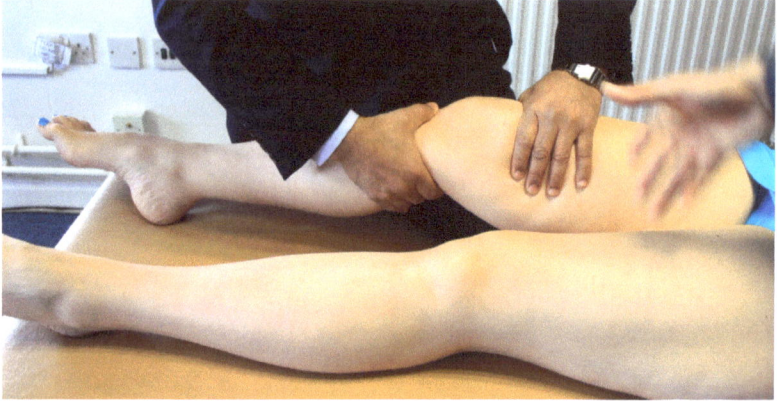

PCL – AP glide, Sag test, Quadriceps active test

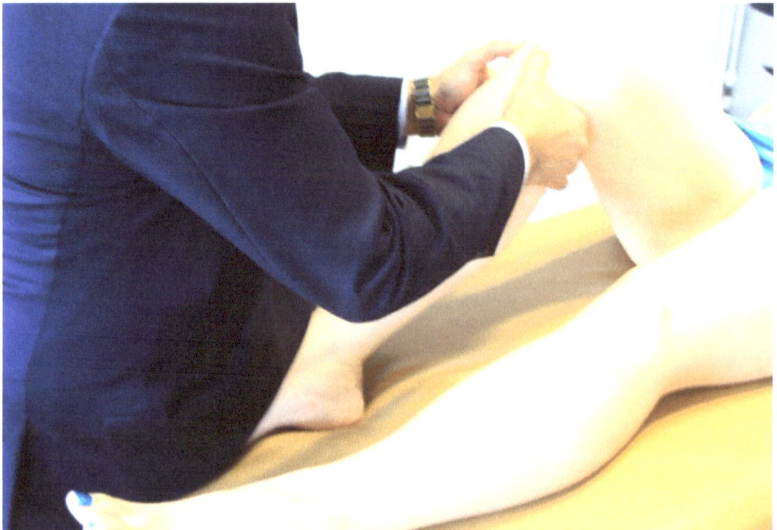

PLC – Dial test, Hughston's posteromedial/posterolateral drawer test, Reverse pivot shift, look for Varus recurvatum

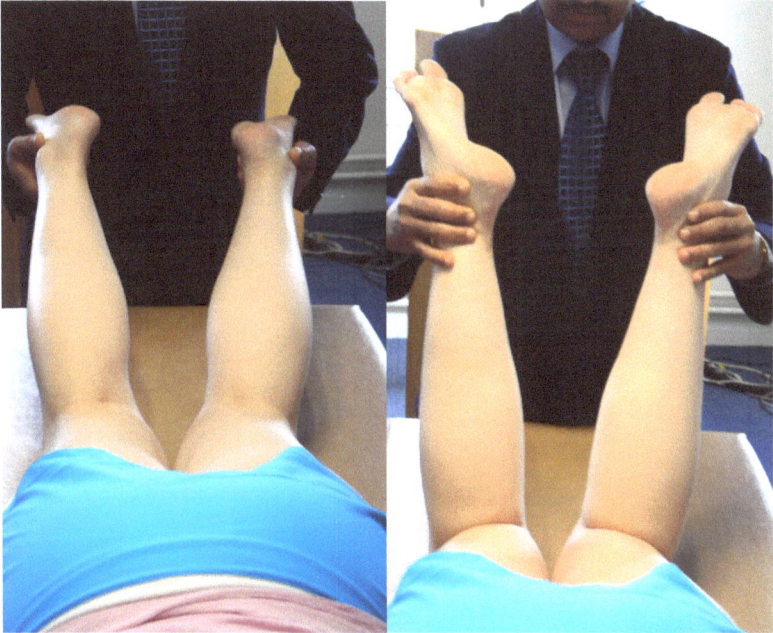

Patella – Apprehension test, Assess femoral and tibial rotation

Examine the neurovascular status of lower limb

Finally mention to examine hip and ankle.

Shoulder examination

Patient undresses up to waist, males completely, female patient with bra can move strap.

Look

look for prominence, scars, swelling, muscle wasting

Front
- Neck position
- SC Joint
- Clavicle
- AC Joint

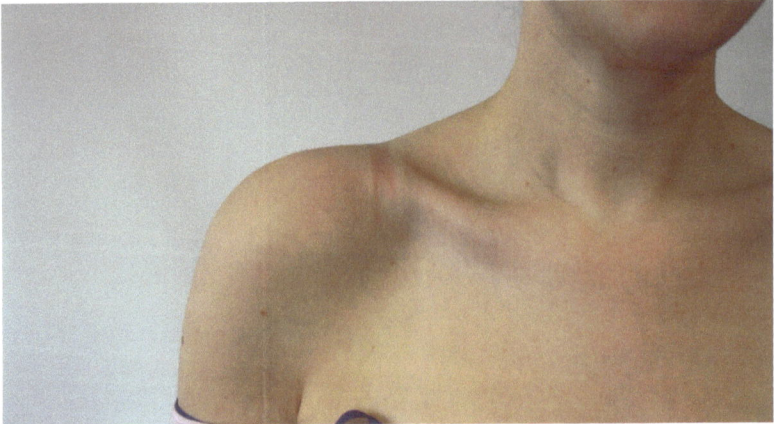

Side
- Deltoid contour
- Scar

Back
- Neck position

- Scapular position
- SS Fossa
- IS Fossa

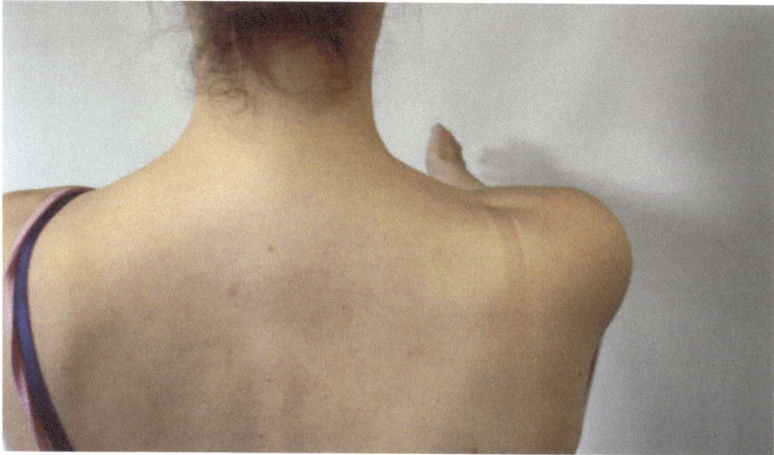

Feel

Feel for tenderness, sensitivity and skin mobility

- SC joint/AC joint
- Clavicle / Coracoid
- Tuberosities / Intertubercular groove
- Lateral border of acromion / Scapular spine
- SS/IS fossa / Scapula medial border

Move

- Explain and show to the patient
- Stay behind the patient
- Active movement first and then passive movements
- Scapulothoracic rhythm

Forward Flexion

Elevation

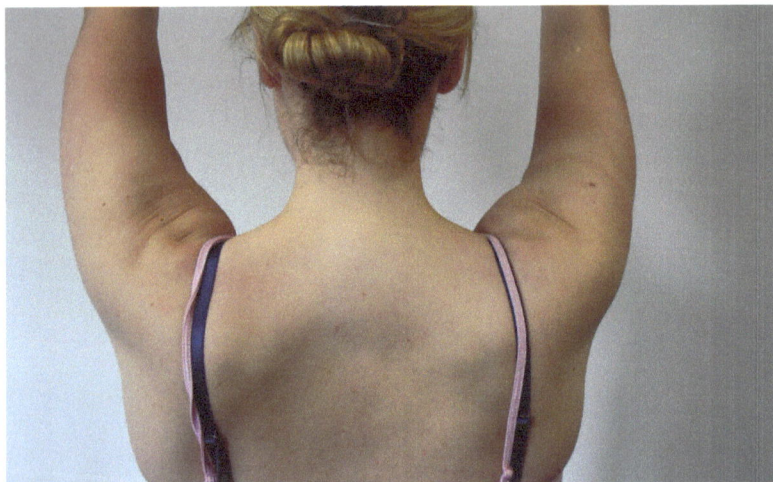

Abduction

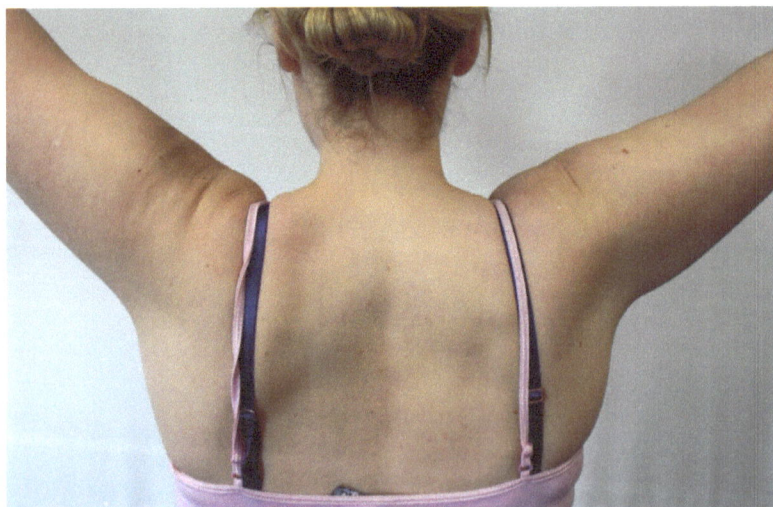

External Rotation

Internal Rotation

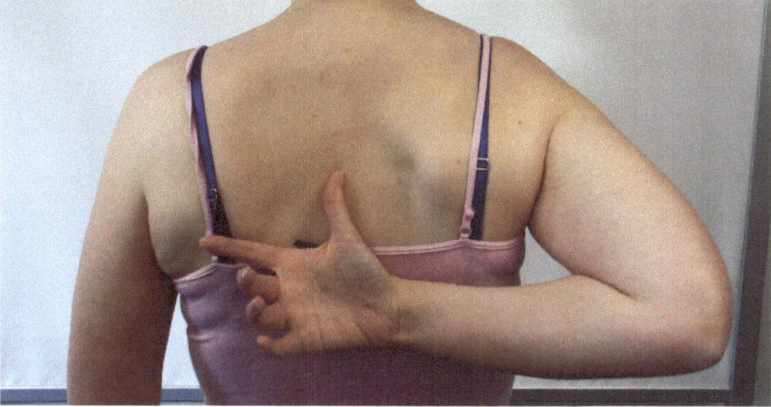

Special Test

Impingement

- Neer's Sign
- Hawkins-Kennedy test

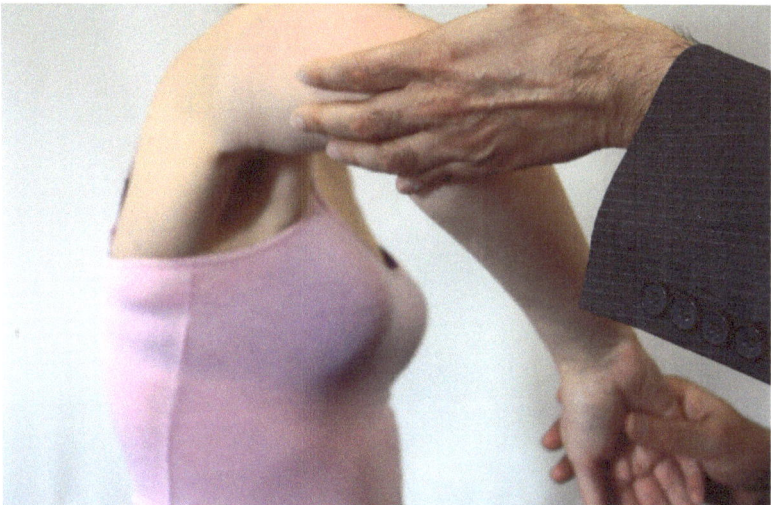

AC Joint pathology

- Scarf test (Cross-arm adduction with elbow flexed or extended)

Frozen Shoulder

- Loss of External Rotation with normal Radiographs

Rotator Cuff Pathology

- Empty Can test - Supraspinatus
- External Rotation Lag Sign - Infraspinatus
- Gerber's Lift-Off Test - Subscapularis

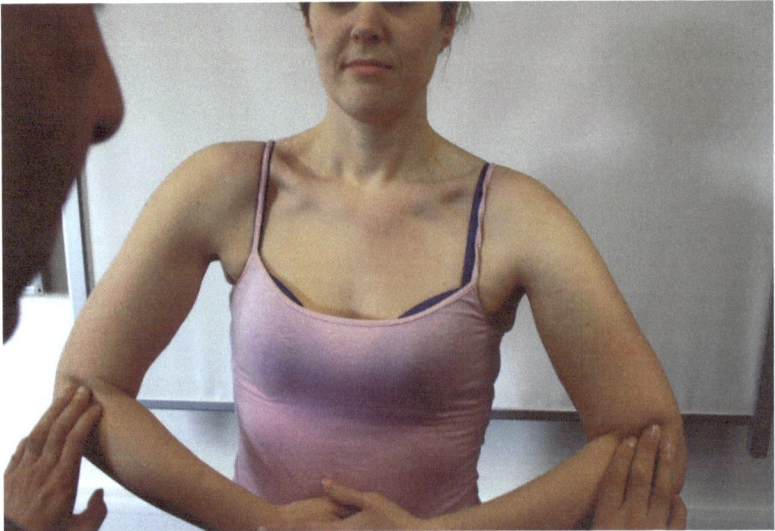

Massive Cuff Tear

- Hornblower's sign
- The Dropping Sign

Instability

- Anterior Apprehension test
- Anterior Drawer Test
- Jobe Relocation test
- Load and Shift Test
- Sulcus test

SLAP Lesions

- O'Brien test

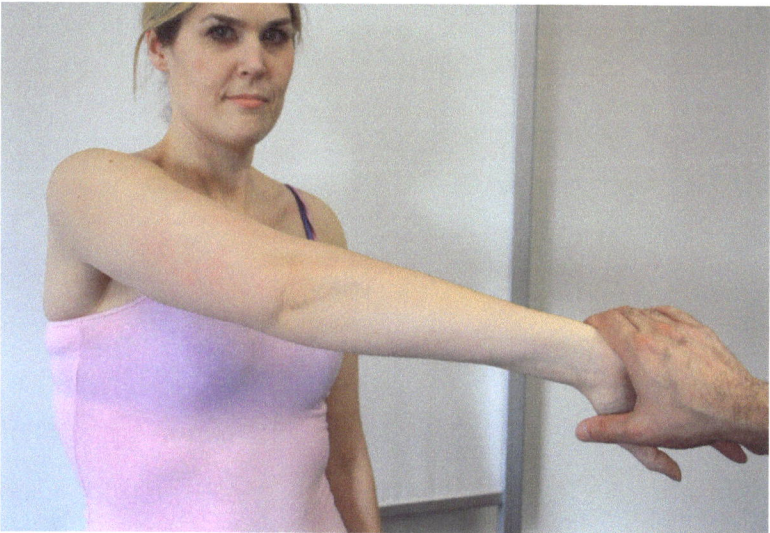

LHB – Long Head of Biceps Pathology

- Yergasons Test
- Speed's Test

Spine examinaion

In spine cases usually hints for diagnosis are in the question therefore it is important to listen to the examiner or carefully read the GP letter.

The common cases will be Spinal stenosis/Back pain, Myelopathy and Scoliosis.

Introduce yourself to the patient; ask permission for the examination.

Look around for walking aid, prosthesis; ask the patient to stand. The patient should be undressed.

Standing

Look

Front
- Sagittal balance
- Shoulder asymmetry
- Pelvic asymmetry

Back
- Spinal curve
- Apex right or left
- Rib hump
- Dimple, nevi, hairy patches, scar

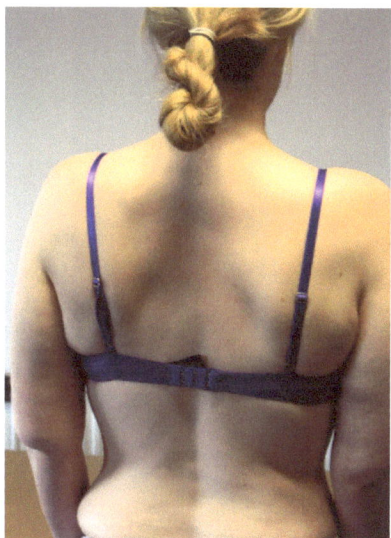

Side

- Normal curvatures of the spine.
- This is cervical lordosis, thoracic kyphosis and lumbar lordosis.

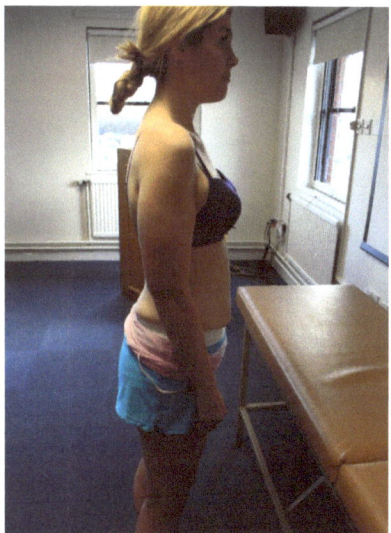

Feel

- Spinous process
- Paraspinal muscles
- Sacroiliac joints

Move

Cervical spine

- *Flexion* - Touch your chin to your chest

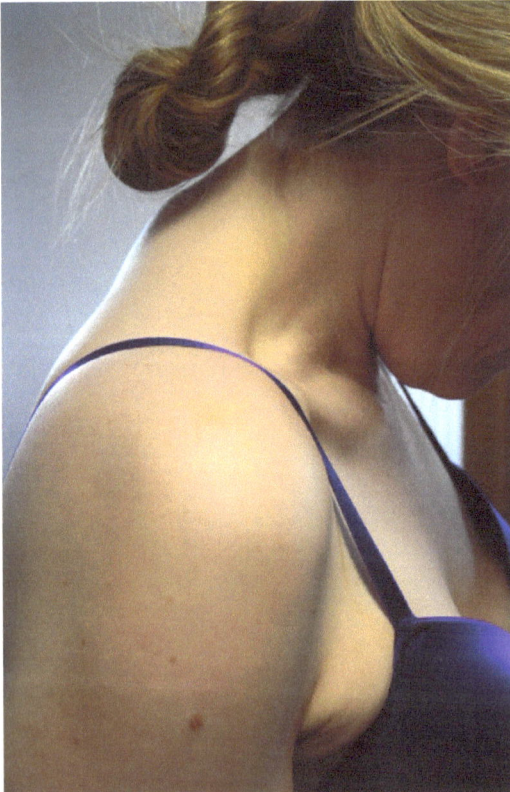

- *Extension - Look at the ceiling*

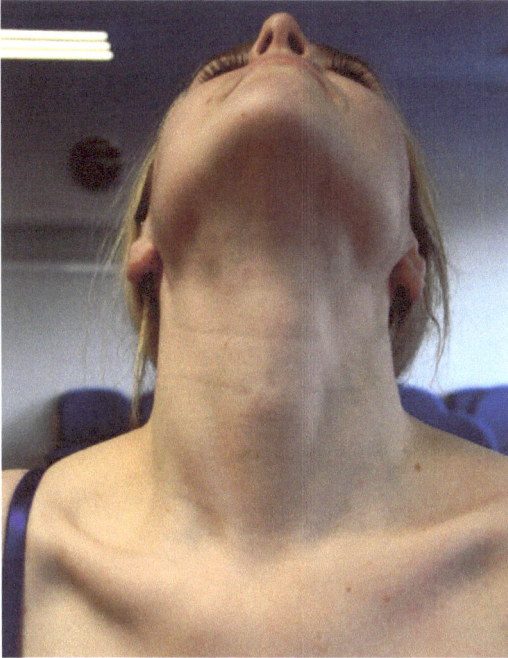

- *Lateral Flexion* - Touch your ear to your shoulder

- *Rotation* - Look at your shoulder

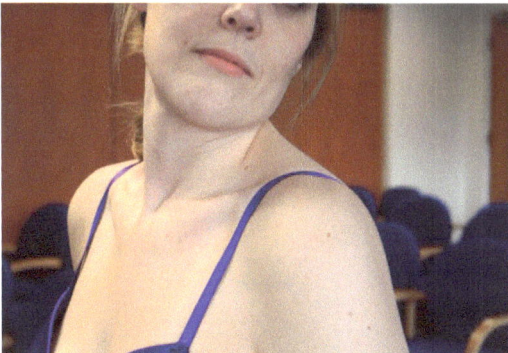

Thoracic spine

- Rotation
- Adam test

Lumbar spine

- Flexion
- Extension
- Lateral Bending
- Rotation

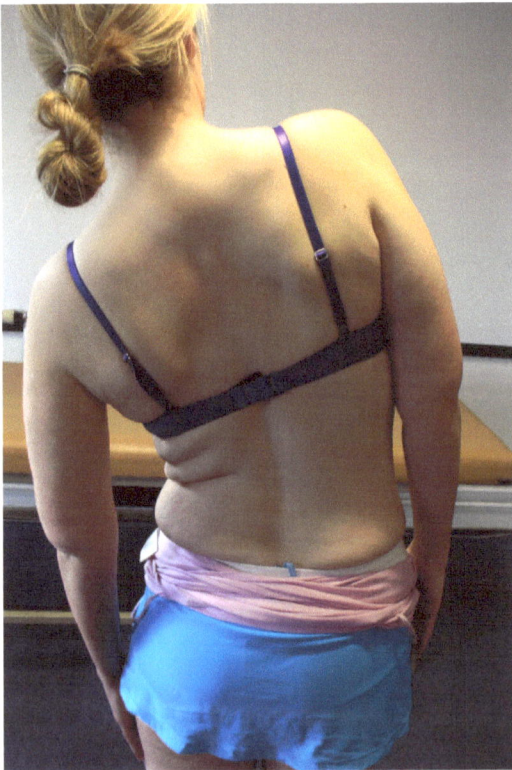

Shober test

Sitting

Back
- Structural or
- Functional
- In functional scoliosis curve disappears on sitting down

Lying Down

SLR

Neurological Examination

Sensation

Ask the patient to close their eyes and tell you when they feel you touching them.

Use a light touch of the finger, have a system in mind with a logical progression sequential dermatome mapping.

Note any areas of hypoaesthesia or dysaesthesia.

Tone

This is the resistance felt when joint is passively moved. Make sure patient is fully relaxed during examination.

Hypertonia is a sign of Upper Motor Neurone Lesion.

Hypotonia is found in Lower Motor Neurone Lesion.

Power

Use MRC grading system when describing power.

Get patient to contract the muscle group being tested and then you try to overpower that group.

Reflexes

- Biceps
- Triceps
- Brachioradialis
- Abdominal
- Knee
- Ankle

Special Test

Femoral stretch

Sciatic stretch

Sacroiliac joint
- Tenderness
- FABER Test
- Gaenslen Test

Vascular Exam

Spinal Stenosis

After spine examination assess lower limb neurological examination

Sensation

- L2: upper thigh
- L3: knee
- L4: medial aspect of the leg
- L5: lateral aspect of the leg, medial side of the dorsum of the foot
- S1: lateral aspect of the foot, the heel and most of the sole
- S2: posterior aspect of the thigh
- S3-S5: concentric rings around the anus, the outermost of which is S3

Tone

Make sure patient is fully relaxed.

This is the resistance felt when joint is moved passively through its normal range of movement.

Power

Test one muscle group for each function

- L2, L3: hip flexion and internal rotation
- L4, L5: hip extension and external rotation
- L3, L4: knee extension
- L5, S1: knee flexion
- L4, L5: ankle dorsiflexion
- S1, S2: ankle plantar flexion

- L4: ankle inversion
- L5, S1: ankle eversion

Reflexes

- Knee
- Ankle

Special test

- SLR
- Femoral stretch
- Sciatic Stretch

Cervical Radiculopathy

Neurological features associated with cervical radiculopathy

C5 nerve root:
- Muscle weakness: shoulder abduction and flexion/elbow flexion
- Reflex changes: biceps
- Sensory changes: lateral arm

C6 nerve root:
- Muscle weakness: elbow flexion/wrist extension
- Reflex changes: biceps/supinator
- Sensory changes: lateral forearm, thumb, index finger

C7 nerve root:
- Muscle weakness: elbow extension, wrist flexion, finger extension
- Reflex changes: triceps
- Sensory changes: middle finger

C8 nerve root:
- Muscle weakness: finger flexion
- Reflex changes: none
- Sensory changes: medial side lower forearm, ring and little finger

T1 nerve root:
- Muscle weakness: finger abduction and adduction
- Reflex changes: none
- Sensory changes: medial side upper arm/lower arm.

Myelopathy

Gait

- Romberg test

C spine

- Look
- Feel
- Move

Upper limb neurology

- Sensation
- Tone
- Motor
- Reflexes

Abdominal reflexes

Lower limb neurology

- Sensation
- Tone
- Motor
- Reflexes

Upper motor neuron signs –

- Increased tone
- Decreased power
- Hoffman's sign

- Inverted radial reflex
- Clonus

Vascular examination

Scoliosis

Usually short case but can be a long case; in short case child or adolescent is sitting and candidate is asked to be examined.

Look around for any braces, walking aid, orthotics.

Ask patient to stand; introduce yourself and explain to him or her that you are going to examine them.

Standing

Look

Front
- Sagittal balance
- Shoulder asymmetry
- Pelvic asymmetry

Back
- Spinal curve
- Apex right or left
- Rib hump
- Dimple, nevi, hairy patches, scar

Sitting

Back
- Structural or
- Functional
- In functional scoliosis curve disappears on sitting down

Neurological Examination

Special test

- Adam's forward bending test

Brachial Plexus Examination

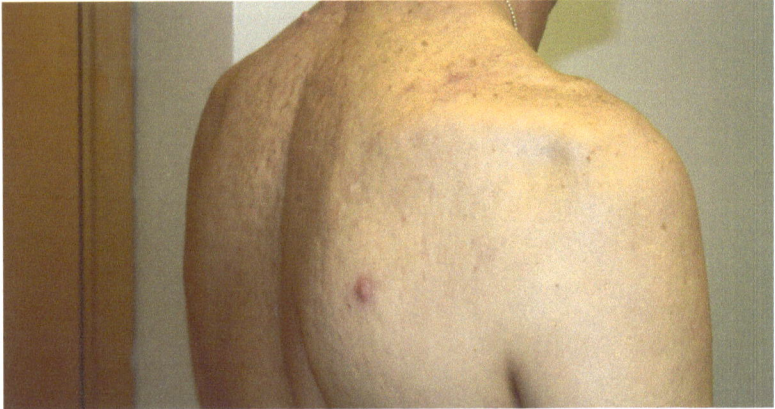

In Brachial plexus, the whole purpose of the examination is to determine the level of the lesion, the extent of the injury, the presence of any poor prognostic sign and to map out sensory deficit and motor function loss. After finishing the BP exam candidates should be able to answer which nerve root, cord or nerve is involved.

Look

Front

Face

- Horner's syndrome

Shoulder

- Scars

Arm position

- adducted / abduction
- internal / external rotation
- Forearm – pronation / supination
- Wrist – flexed / extended
- Fingers – position of MCPJ / IPJ

Side

Wasting

Scapula

- Winging

Feel

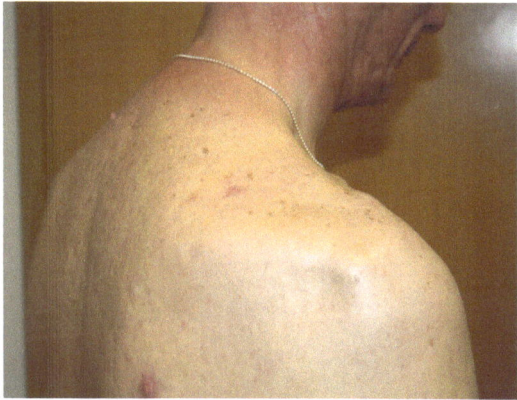

Sensory
- Dermatomes sensation
- Peripheral nerves

Move

Assess the myotomes' power

Shoulder

Back
- Shrug – Trapezius, Levator scapulae
- Brace back – Rhomboids
- Scapula winging – Serratus Anterior

Side

- Deltoid
- Pact. Major
- Latis. Dorsi

Front

- Supraspinatus
- Infraspinatus
- Subscapularis

Elbow

- Biceps
- Triceps

Wrist

- Flexion
- Extension

Hand

- Flexion
- Abduction

Bad prognostic signs

- Horner's syndrome
- Pre-ganglionic injuries – involvement of Rhomboids and Serratus Anterior
- Painful anaesthetic limb

Neurological Features

C5 nerve root:
- Muscle weakness: shoulder abduction and flexion/elbow flexion
- Reflex changes: biceps
- Sensory changes: lateral arm

C6 nerve root:
- Muscle weakness: elbow flexion/wrist extension
- Reflex changes: biceps/supinator
- Sensory changes: lateral forearm, thumb, index finger

C7 nerve root:
- Muscle weakness: elbow extension, wrist flexion, finger extension
- Reflex changes: triceps
- Sensory changes: middle finger

C8 nerve root:
- Muscle weakness: finger flexion
- Reflex changes: none
- Sensory changes: medial side lower forearm, ring and little finger

T1 nerve root:
- Muscle weakness: finger abduction and adduction
- Reflex changes: none
- Sensory changes: medial side upper arm/lower arm.

Child examination

Cerebral Palsy

May be a long case – it is distressing but if you have a system you will sail through.

Try to keep your composure and start in a systematic way.

General

Sitting

Standing

Walking

Lying down on couch

- Supine
- Lateral position
- Prone

General Examination

Look around and comment on presence of wheelchair, walking aids, braces and orthotics.

Patient posture and any pattern of movements (athetoid, spastic) and involvement of whole or part of the body, eg monoplegic, hemiplegic or paraplegic. Is the patient using arms and legs? Do they look paralysed?

Standing

Ask if the patient is able to stand.

Look

Front
- Obvious deformity
- Joint contracture

Back
- Scoliosis
- Adam's test

Side
- Posture in Sagittal plane
- Joint contracture
- Flexion at hips, knee or ankle

If pelvic obliquity and limb length discrepancy use block to confirm

Walking

This is the major part and candidate can secure extra marks. Sometimes walking video of child is shown in paediatric viva.

Just describe the gait in three planes; don't look for fancy words – use simple plain English to describe walking in three planes, ie sagittal, transverse and coronal plane.

Sitting

If the patient can't stand, examine in sitting position on the couch

Look for

- shoulder asymmetry
- pelvic obliquity
- pressure areas
- spine from behind

Supine

Lay down patient on patient on the couch with knee to the end and legs hanging over end of couch.

Start the lower leg examination.

Hips
- Thomas's test for fixed flexion contracture of hips
- Test abduction of the hips
- External and internal rotation of the hips with knee flexed

Knees
- Extension and flexion active and passive
- Popliteal angle test

For hamstring tightness, flex hip to 90 degrees, attempt to extend the knee, the popliteal angle is that in front of knee.

Ankle
- Silverskiold's test for Achilles tendon tightness

Feet
- Feet deformities, whether fixed or flexible

Lateral Position

- Ober's test
- Abductor power

Prone Position

- Duncan Ely test
- Staheli's rotational profile test
- Brachial Plexus Examination

Notes

Short cases

Short Cases

There are three short cases for upper limb and three for lower limb.

Allow five minutes for each case and whilst walking to see the next case there are one or two questions examiners can ask about the last case.

Follow the routine during the short cases also, ie:

Look

Feel

Move

Special tests

When you know the case say the spot diagnosis first and start describing beginning with 'look' first.

Upper limb short cases

Dupuytren's Contracture

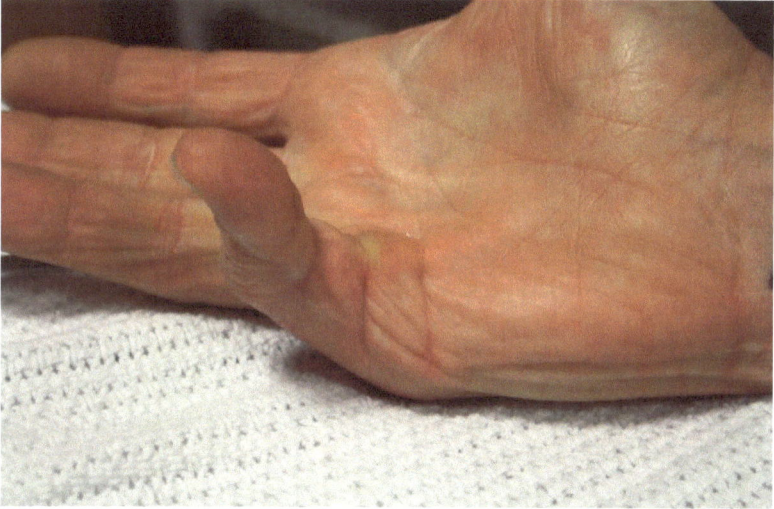

Look

Front
- Skin pits, nodules, cords, finger deformity at MCPH & PIPJ

Back
- Garrod's pads
- Other sites: hand, sole, ask for genitalia

Feel

- Feel cords with index finger from radial to ulnar side, proximal to distal
- Sensation for each side of digital nerve
- Circulation – Digital Allen's test

Move

- Mass movements active and passive
- Individual finger movement, describe flexion contracture at MCPJ & PIPJ

Special test

Hueston's tabletop test

Digital Allen's test

Hand function

- Key grip
- Precision grip
- Tripod grip
- Hook grip
- Power grip

First CMC joint arthritis

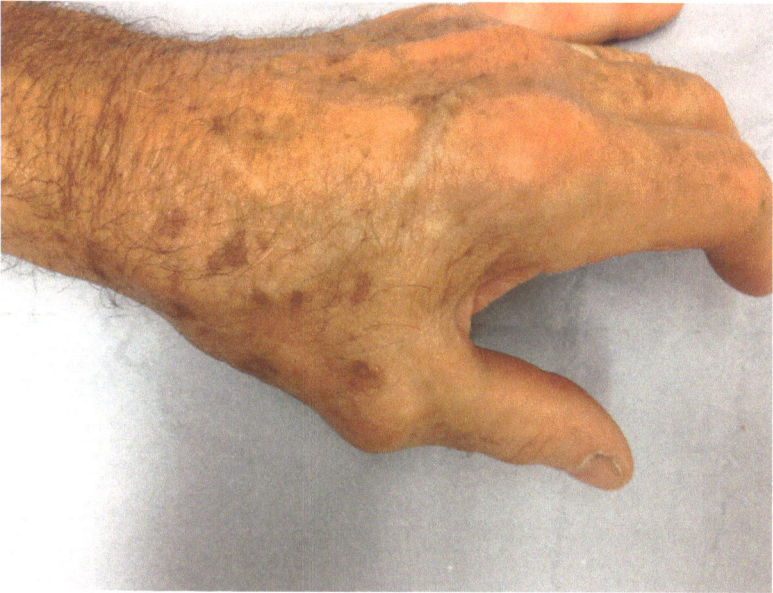

Look

- Prominent 1st MC base – Shoulder sign
- Thinner muscle wasting
- MCP Joint hyperextension
- First web space adduction contracture

Back

- First dorsal interosseous wasting
- Skin changes over CMC joints, eg depigmentation due to steroid injections

Feel

- Tenderness localisation from proximal to distal
- for De Quervain's disease, CMCJ, MCPJ & STT
- Distal Neurovascular status

Move

- Thumb movements active/passive at CMCJ & MCPJ
- Finger movement to exclude trigger finger
- Wrist and forearm movement

Special test

Axial grind test (axial compression and rotation – painful)

Crank test (axial compression and Flexion/Extension – painful)

Hand function

- Key grip
- Precision grip
- Tripod grip
- Hook grip
- Power grip

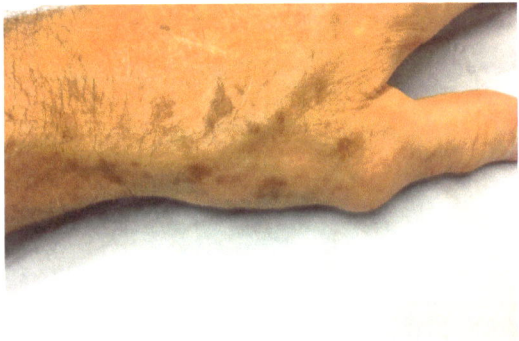

Exclude associated Carpal Tunnel Syndrome and Trigger fingers.

Carpal Tunnel Syndrome

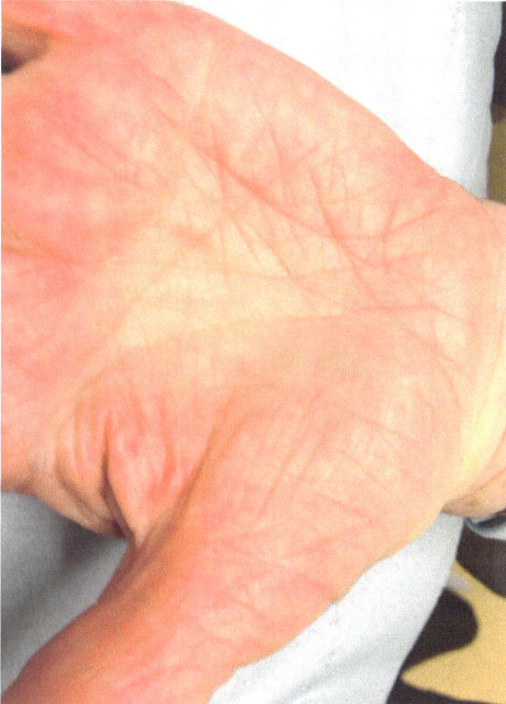

Look

- Scar
- Thinner Wasting (abductor Pollicis Brevis)
- Trophic changes over median nerve distribution

Feel

- Sensation (superficial branch over thinner muscles and radial three digits)

- Volar aspect of index finger
- Over thinner eminence
- Scar tenderness

Motor

- Abductor Pollicis Brevis (APB)
- Flexor digitorum superficial (FDS)
- Radial half of Flexor digitorum profundus (FDP)
- Flexor Pollicis longus (FPL)

Move

- Wrist and hand movement

Special test

Phalen's test

Durkan's test

Tinel's sign

Test for Donors

Palmaris Longus

Extensor Indicis Proprius

Abductor digiti Minimi

Rheumatoid hand

Bilateral symmetrical polyarthropathy involving small joint of the hand and wrist – probably inflammatory. I would like to start the examination from neck, shoulder and elbow but for this exam I will concentrate on the hand and wrist.

Look

Dorsal aspect

- Proximal to distal
- Ulnar to radial

Side

Volar aspect

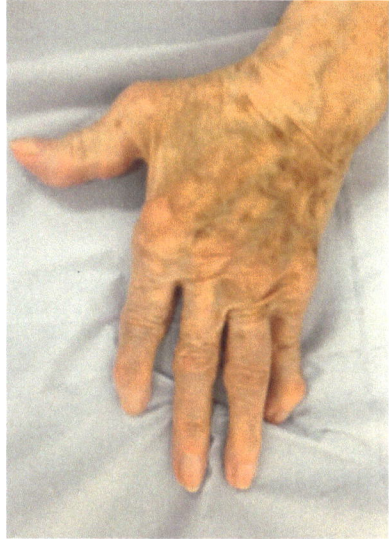

- Elbow – rheumatoid nodule ulnar border
- Wrist – swelling and ulnar head
- MCPJ – swelling/subluxation/ulnar deviation
- Finger and thumb – deformity swan neck/boutonniere

Feel

- Swelling
- Deformity, correctable or not
- Warmth
- Pain

Move

(Neck, shoulder, elbow)

- Wrist
- Thumb and fingers

Special test

- Piano key test
- Wrist flexion and extension

Ganglion

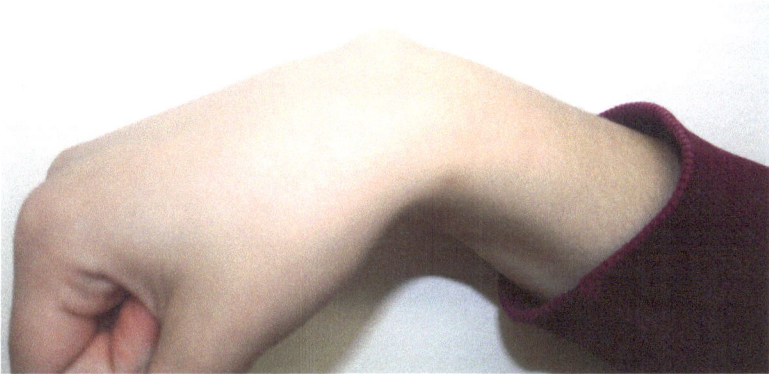

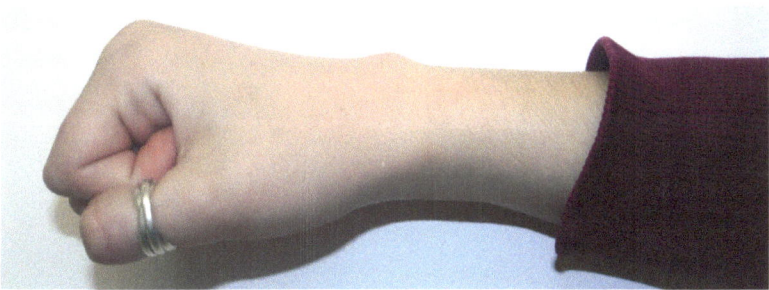

Dorsal

- Mobile skin
- Increase size in flexion
- Range of wrist movement
- Transillumination

Kirk Watson to check scapholunate instability

Volar

Allen test for vascular patency of radial and ulnar artery.

Mucous cyst

- Skin mobility
- Nail ridges
- OA of DIP joints

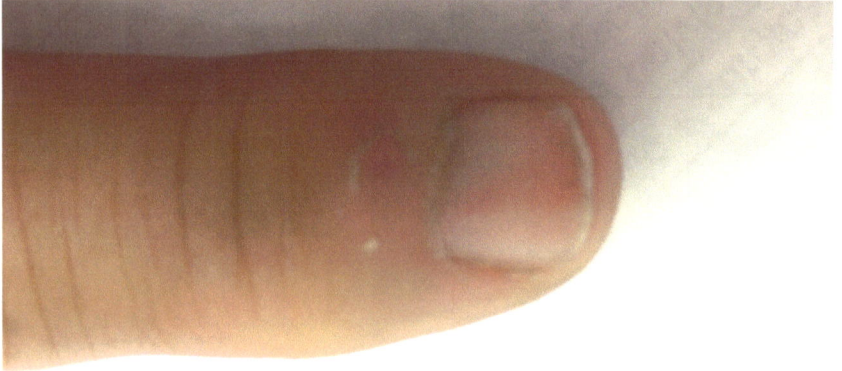

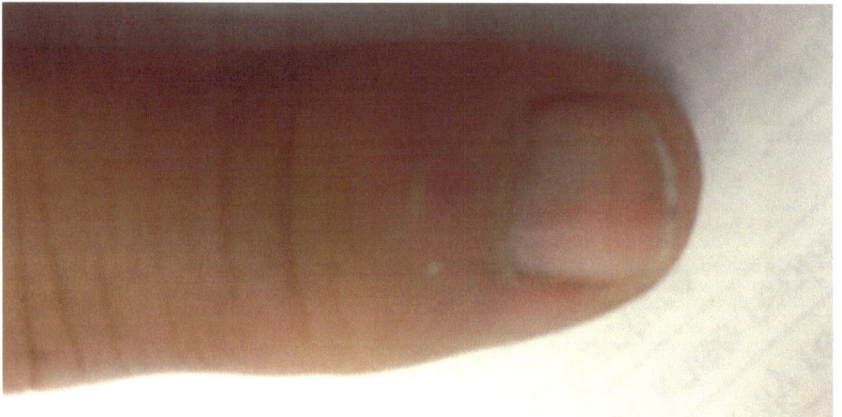

Ulnar Nerve

Look

- Thinner eminence
- Intrinsic muscle wasting /guttering
- Clawing
- Wartenberg sign
- Elbow scar

Feel

Tinel's sign
Ulnar nerve
subluxation

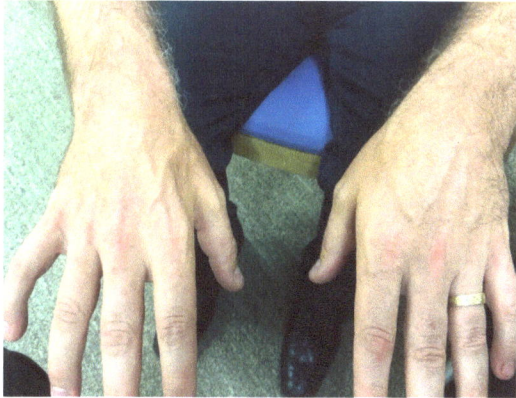

Sensory

- Little finger/ index finger comparison
- Hypothenar / Dorsal side of hand ulnar aspect comparison

Motor

- FCU
- Froment test
- Card test

Provocative test

- Elbow flexion for 30 seconds

Radial Nerve / PIN

Look

- Drop wrist
- Elbow radial side wasting

Feel

Sensory

- Dorsum of first web (presence in PIN Palsy)

Motor

- Triceps, Brachioradialis, ECRL (spared in PIN palsy)
- ECRB, EDC, EIP, EDM, EPL, APL, EPB

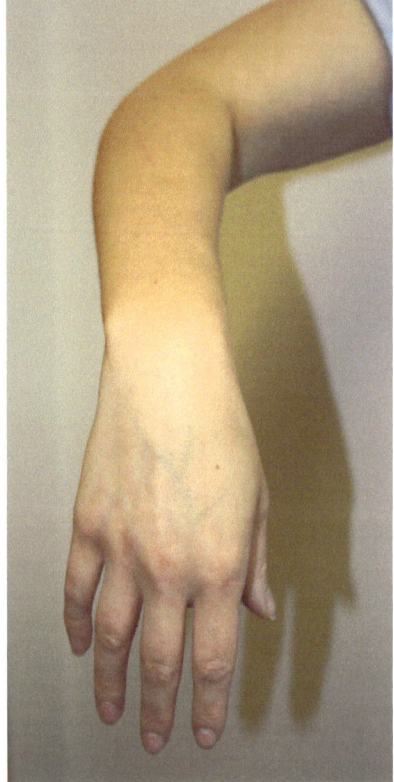

Move

- Wrist goes in radial deviation – PIN Palsy
- Wrist drop Radial Palsy

Shoulder Arthrodesis

Look

- Scar – multiple scar or long scars from neck to shoulder
- Deltoid Contour – wasting of deltoid and trapezius

Feel

- Scar for tenderness
- Hypersensitivity
- Neurovascular status of upper limb

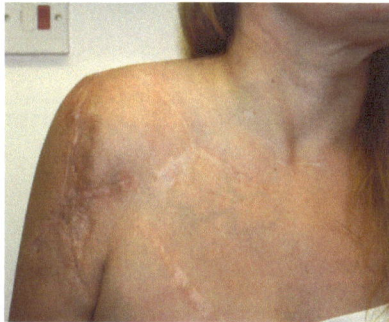

Move

Isolate glenohumeral from scapulothoracic movements

Glenohumeral joint

- Hold scapula – with arm abduction scapula moves with it (normally scapula starts moving after 60 degrees)

Special test

Upper limb functional assessment

- Ability to reach mouth
- Ability to reach bottom

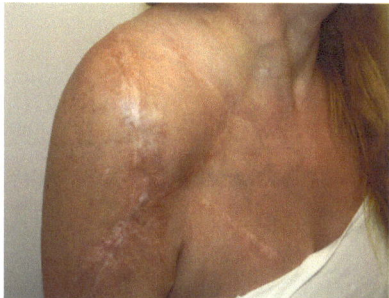

Sprengel Deformity

Look

From front, side and back for:

Unilateral or bilateral.
If bilateral then high shoulders – shoulder starts after head; there is no distinction of neck in-between.

Position of scapula, fully developed or hypoplastic

Scar
- on neck
- on chest
- on abdomen

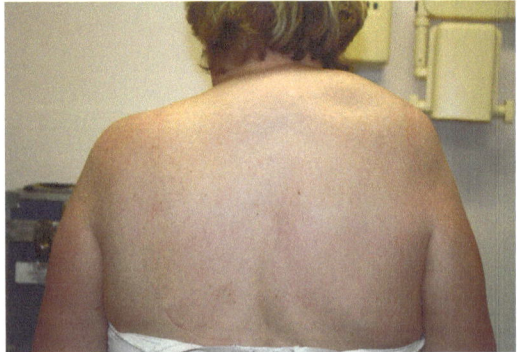

Feel

- scar
- scapula
- check connection between scapula and neck, ie fibrous, bony

Move

Scapulothoracic rhythm

- describe scapula movement in relation to shoulder movement

Special tests

- Look for sign of previous surgery – cardiac, renal problem
- Neurovascular examination of upper limb

Associations

- Klippel-Feil syndrome
- Short web neck
- Low hair line
- Stiff neck – decreased ROM
- Cardiac anomalies
- Renal anomalies

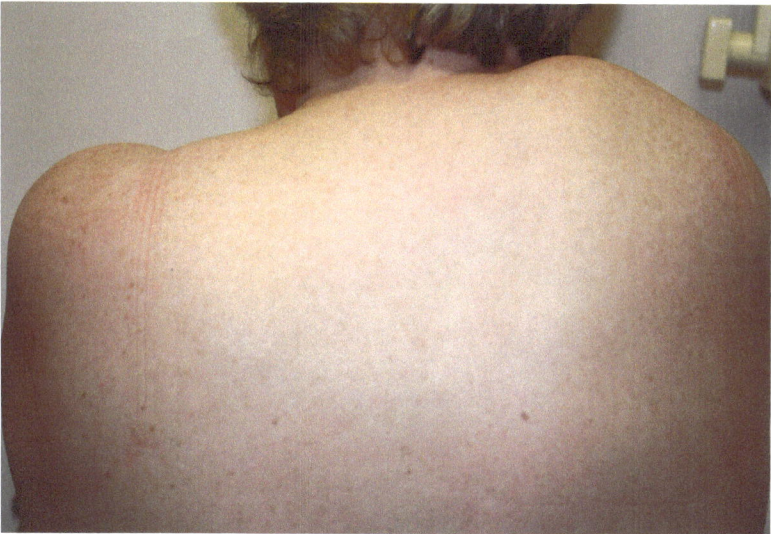

Notes

Lower limb short cases

Hallux valgus

Look for shoe, describe wear pattern and orthosis

Look

Standing

Front
- Shoes/stick/orthotics
- Hallux valgus big toe
- Medial bunion
- Lesser toe deformity
- Scars
- Swelling

Side
- Arches
- Scar/swelling
- Rotational deformity of the toes

Back
- Spine
- Calf
- Heel

Sitting

Sole
- Callosity
- Scar

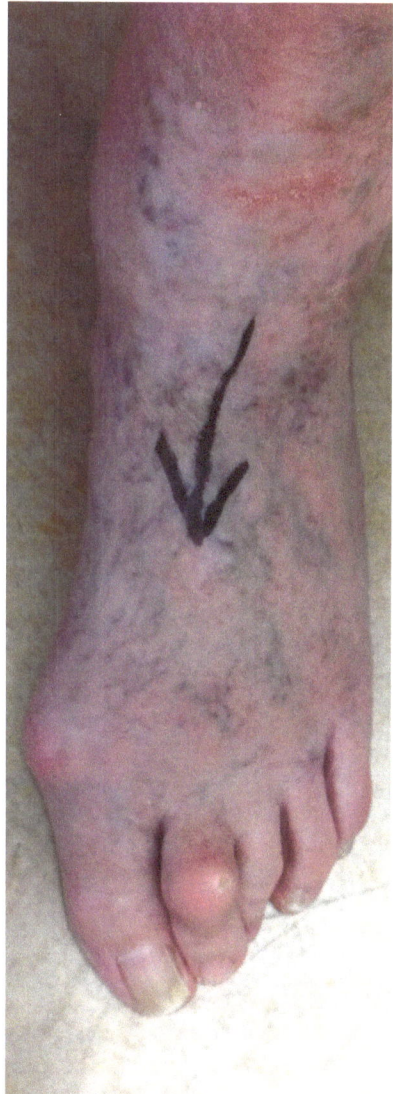

Gait

- Phases of gait

Feel

- Correctable/partial correctable deformities
- MTPJ (1st) lesser MTPJ, TMT
- Tenderness
- Neurovascular status

Move

- Dorsal/plantar flexion IP
- Midfoot
- Ankle

Special test

- Tip toe
- Achilles tightness Silfverskiold test

Key facts

Skin condition

DCN integrity

Vascularity

Degenerative disease, eg OA

Pronation

Mid foot instability

Footwear

Hallux rigidus

Look

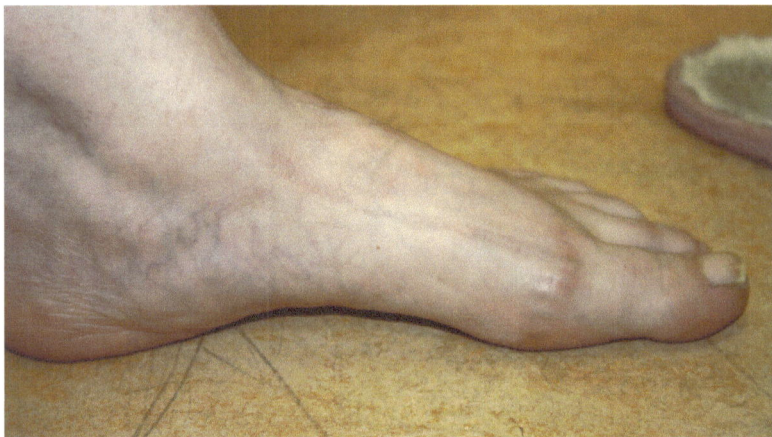

Front
- Shoes/stick/orthotics
- Dorsal bunion
- Lesion toes

Side
- Prominence over the MTPJ
- Longitudinal arch
- Rotational deformity

Back
- Spine/calf/heel

Sole
- Callosity
- Scar

Feel

- Tenderness
- Neurovascular status

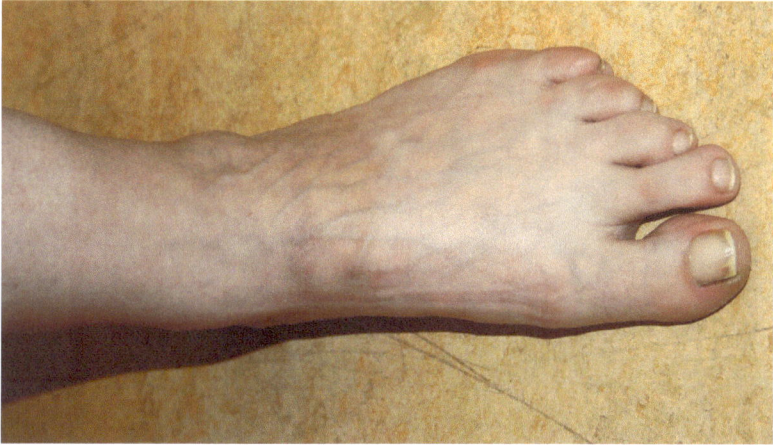

Move

- MTP 1st lesser toes
- IPJ
- TMTs
- Ankle

Key Facts

IP Joint condition

Lesser Toes

Cavus foot

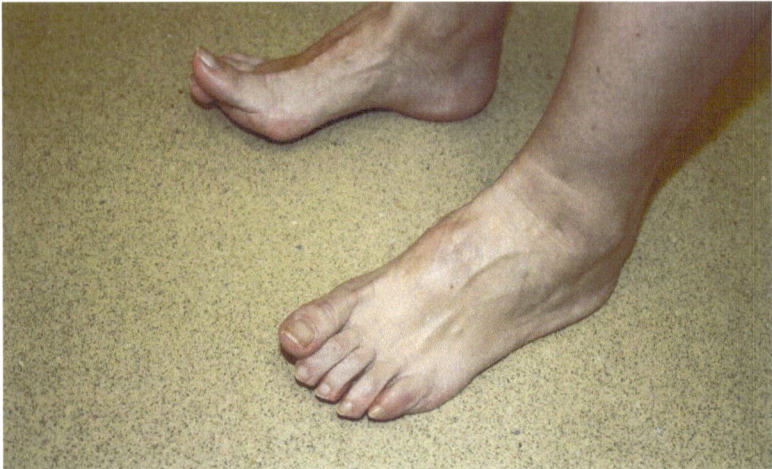

Look

- Spine
- Calf
- Hands
- Shoes

Front
- Claw toes
- Callosities over PIPJ and lateral border
- Medial arch height

Back
- Varus – no change on tip toe
- Spine
- Calf

Sole
- Callosities

Feel

- Toes flexible/stiff
- Toes instability
- Tendon – tib anterior, peroneus longus, Achilles tendon

Neurology

- Ankle Jerk

Special test

- Coleman block test

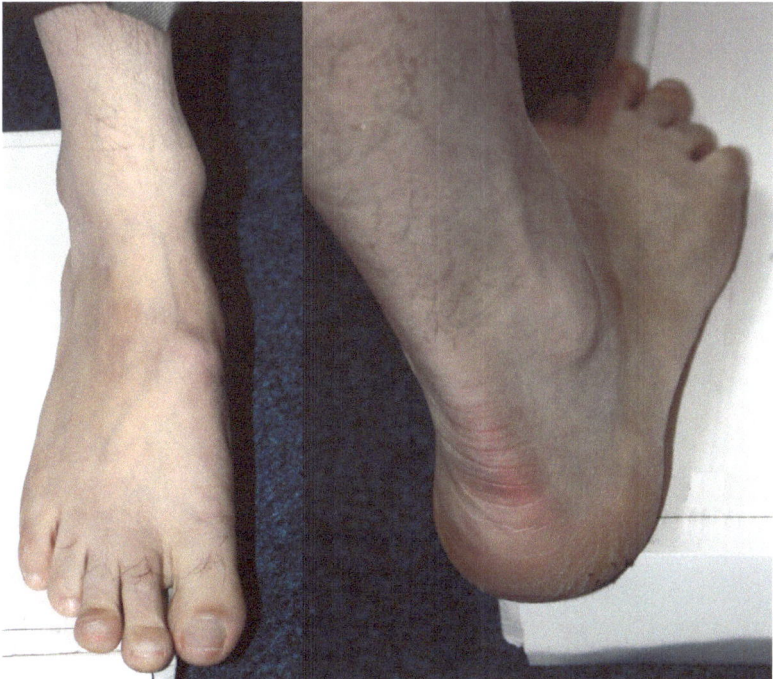

Key Facts

Skin

Spine

Hand

Neurovascular status

Tibialis Posterior Deficiency

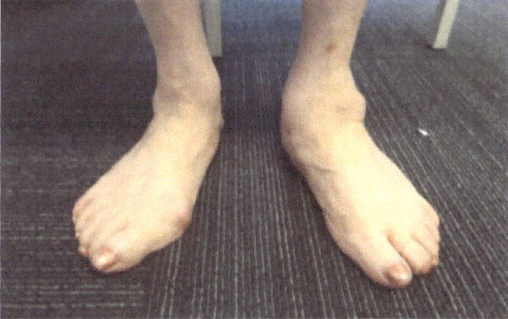

Look

Front
- Shoes/stick/orthotics
- Stance
- Arches
- Forefoot
- Midfoot

Side
- Swelling around medial malleolus

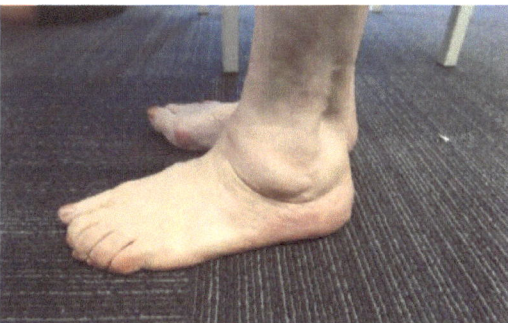

Back

- Spine
- Calf
- Heel Valgus
- Too many toes sign

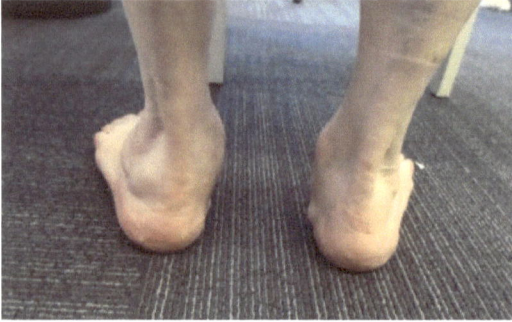

Sole

- Swelling
- Callosity

Walk

- Gait

Feel

- Tenderness
- Tibialis posterior
- FHL, FDL, Achilles tendon
- Neurovascular status

Move

- Forefoot
- Ankle
- Subtalar

Special test

- Tip toes – double/single

Key Fact

Fibular impingement

Correctable, ie Flexible / Fixed

Achilles tendon

Look

- Front
- Side
- Back
- Sole

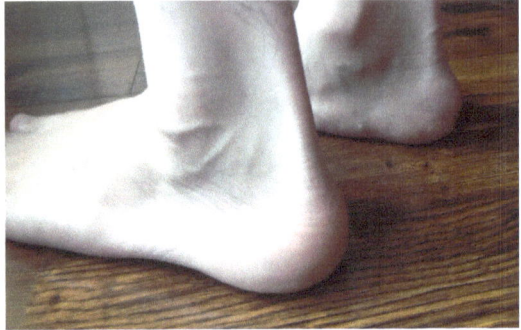

Walk

- Tip toes

Feel

- Tenderness
- Achilles tendon
- Neurovascular status

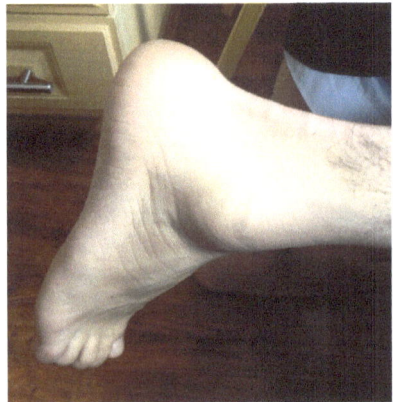

Move

- Forefoot, midfoot, ankle, ST
- No active plantar flexion

Special test

- Thompson test (Simmonds test)
- Calf squeeze test Ankle Arthrodesis

Ankle Arthrodesis

Look

- Shoes' wear pattern
- Gait – no initial contact and no rockers
- Chronic changes over distal leg and foot (CRPS)

Front
- Scar
- Swelling
- Prominent tendon

Side
- Scar
- Swelling
- Tendons

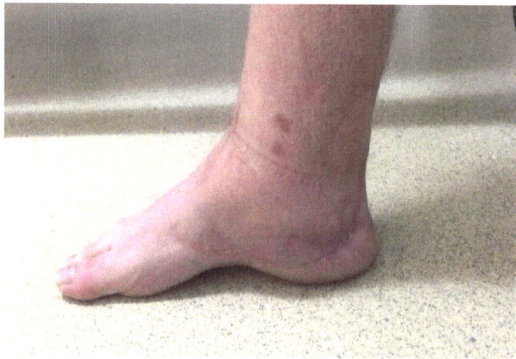

Back
- Scar
- Swelling
- Achilles tendon

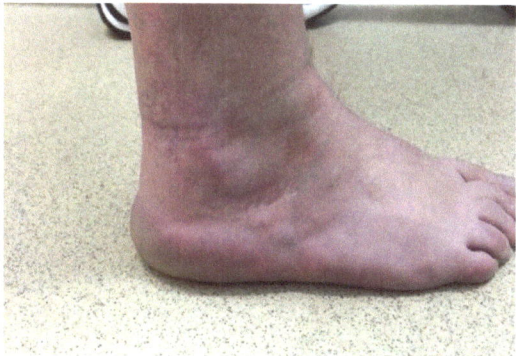

Feel

For temperature, tenderness and Neurovascular status distally

- Scar
- Joint Line

- Tendon around peroneals, Achilles, Tib.Post

Move

No movements at ankle joint

- Subtalar joint
- Midtarsal joint – increased range of movement

Neurovascular status

Describe position of arthrodesis, ie degrees of plantar/dorsal flexion, varus/vagus.

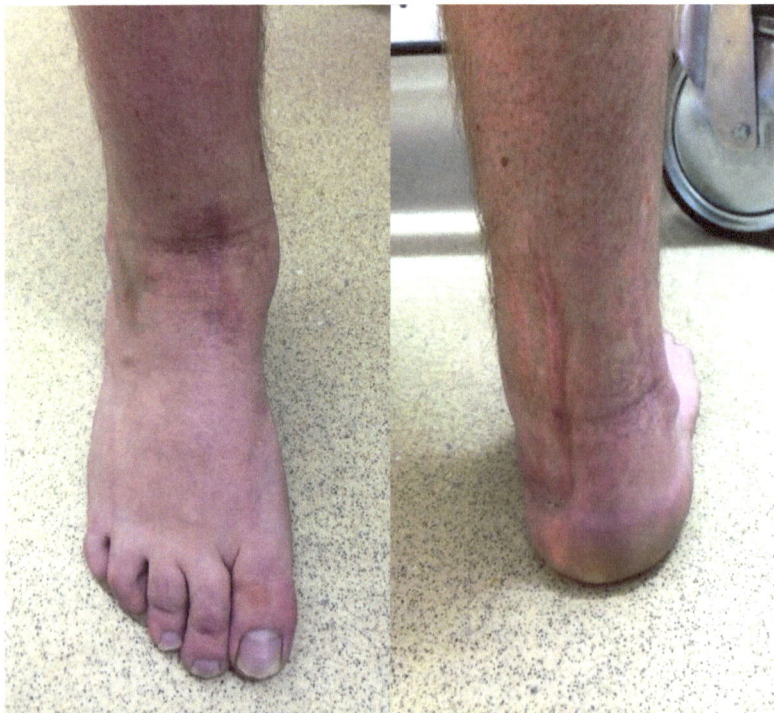

Notes

MRC scale for muscle power

0   No muscle contraction is visible.

1   Muscle contraction is visible but there is no movement of the joint.

2   Active joint movement is possible with gravity eliminated.

3   Movement can overcome gravity but not resistance from the examiner.

4   The muscle group can overcome gravity and move against some resistance from the examiner.

5   Full and normal power against resistance.

To benefit from this book fully, join *orthopaedicstraining.com*

www.ingramcontent.com/pod-product-compliance
Lightning Source LLC
Chambersburg PA
CBHW041311210326
41599CB00003B/65